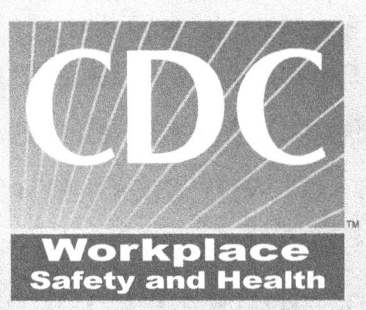

I0426016

Evaluation of Health Concerns in a Public Middle School – Virginia

Elena Page, MD, MPH
Nancy Burton, PhD, MPH, CIH
Melody Kawamoto, MD, MS
R. Todd Niemeier, MS, CIH

Health Hazard Evaluation Report
HETA 2010-0045-3129
June 2011

DEPARTMENT OF HEALTH AND HUMAN SERVICES
Centers for Disease Control and Prevention

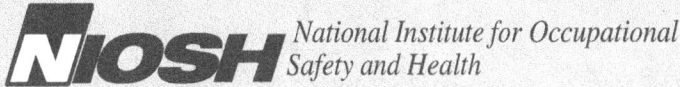

National Institute for Occupational Safety and Health

The employer shall post a copy of this report for a period of 30 calendar days at or near the workplace(s) of affected employees. The employer shall take steps to insure that the posted determinations are not altered, defaced, or covered by other material during such period. [37 FR 23640, November 7, 1972, as amended at 45 FR 2653, January 14, 1980].

CONTENTS

ABBREVIATIONS

ACGIH®	American Conference of Governmental Industrial Hygienists
AIHA	American Industrial Hygiene Association
ANSI	American National Standards Institute
ASHRAE	American Society of Heating, Refrigerating and Air-Conditioning Engineers
CFM	Cubic feet per minute
CFR	Code of Federal Regulations
cm^2	Square centimeter
CO	Carbon monoxide
CO_2	Carbon dioxide
CV	Coefficient of variation
ELISA	Enzyme-linked immunosorbent assay
ERMI	Environmental relative moldiness index
HEPA	High-efficiency particulate air
HHE	Health hazard evaluation
HUD	U.S. Department of Housing and Urban Development
HVAC	Heating, ventilating, and air-conditioning
IEQ	Indoor environmental quality
IOM	Institute of Medicine
Ls^{-1}	Liters per second
MERV	Minimum efficiency reporting value
MSQPCR	Mold-specific quantitative polymerase chain reaction
NAICS	North American Industry Classification System
ND	Not detected
NIOSH	National Institute for Occupational Safety and Health
OEL	Occupational exposure limit
OSHA	Occupational Safety and Health Administration
PEL	Permissible exposure limit
ppm	Parts per million
RH	Relative humidity
µg/g	Microgram per gram
U.S. EPA	United States Environmental Protection Agency
VAV	Variable air volume
VCS	Visual contrast sensitivity
VOC	Volatile organic compound
WHO	World Health Organization

The National Institute for Occupational Safety and Health (NIOSH) received a management request for a health hazard evaluation at a middle school in Virginia. The request was submitted because some employees had concerns about exposure to mold in the school building.

What NIOSH Did

- We evaluated the school in January 2010.

- We interviewed employees. We asked about their work, medical history, and work-related health concerns.

- We looked for signs of water damage and mold in the building and crawl space.

- We looked at the ventilation system design and inspected two of the large units to see how the units were being maintained.

- We checked moisture levels in the walls.

- We collected samples for mold on surfaces and in dust. We also collected dust samples for cat, dog, dust mite, and cockroach allergens.

- We measured carbon dioxide, carbon monoxide, temperature, and relative humidity levels.

What NIOSH Found

- Some employees had been medically evaluated by means of nonstandard medical tests. Their diagnoses and treatments were based on these tests.

- We did not link employees' symptoms and illnesses directly to the conditions found in the school.

- We found that the crawl space under the renovated section of the school was a potential source of mold and dampness.

- The outside soil sloped toward the building, which allowed water to collect at the foundation and would add to the moisture levels in the crawl space.

- Carbon dioxide levels were elevated in some of the classrooms.

- Cat and dog allergens were being brought into the school. The levels that we found could cause health symptoms in allergic individuals.

- The bathrooms in the women's locker room in the new gymnasium had plumbing problems.

What Managers Can Do

- Add crawl space fans to move air from the school into the crawl space. Also add a moisture barrier and seal holes between the crawl space and school.

- Regrade the soil around the building to ensure water does not collect at the foundation and in the crawl space.

- Vacuum the furniture on a regular basis to remove allergens.

- Inspect the ventilation units that serve the classrooms in the renovated section of the building to make sure that adequate amounts of outdoor air are supplied to the occupied areas.

- Identify and fix water leaks in a timely matter.

- Put a no-flush policy into place for feminine hygiene products. This change should address the locker room plumbing issues.

- Create a system in which employees can report building concerns and provide feedback on how issues were resolved.

What Employees Can Do

- Report work-related health concerns to school officials.

- See an experienced occupational medicine physician about health concerns that may be related to work.

- Recognize that some symptoms may not have a medical diagnosis.

- Become active on the indoor environmental quality committee.

SUMMARY

NIOSH investigators evaluated a middle school in Virginia because employees had concerns about exposure to mold in the school. The main problem was that the crawl space under the renovated part of the school was a potential source of mold and dampness because of improper grading and inadequate ventilation. Many of the non-specific symptoms reported, such as sinus problems and headaches, are common among people working in offices and schools, as well as in the general population.

On January 12, 2010, NIOSH received an employer request for an HHE at a middle school in Virginia. The request was made because of staff concerns about exposure to mold in the school building. More than a dozen employees had reported health complaints they thought had been caused by mold since the school underwent renovation in 2006–2007. NIOSH investigators made a site visit on January 27–28, 2010.

We randomly selected 72 (out of 137) employees for confidential medical interviews; 68 were available. In addition, three employees on medical leave and nine employees not on our list were interviewed. We observed workplace conditions and the crawl space beneath the renovated part of the building. We reviewed the HVAC system balancing reports, current HVAC operations, and consultant reports, and we evaluated the functioning of the HVAC system. We measured air pressure differentials between the classrooms and crawl space to determine which direction air was flowing between the two areas. Sticky-tape samples were collected from surfaces for microscopic fungal analysis, and vacuum dust samples were collected from furniture for cat, dog, dust mite, and cockroach allergens. Surfaces were wiped with a Swiffer® sheet and analyzed for the presence of fungal species. A meter was used to measure the interior wall moisture levels. Measurements of CO_2, CO, temperature, and RH were made throughout the workday in the new and renovated classrooms.

Randomly selected school employees had rates of work-related symptoms similar to or below those reported in a study of buildings not known to have IEQ problems and in the general population. Many of the nonspecific symptoms reported, such as sinus problems and headaches, are common among people working in offices and schools, as well as in the general population. More serious health problems reported by some staff are not related to working in the building. The crawl space under the renovated part of the building has a dirt floor with a partial moisture barrier, and the soil slopes toward the foundation instead of away from it, allowing water to enter the crawl space. At the time of our site visit in January 2010, there was no visible mold growth or standing water in the crawl space but there was moisture under the partial moisture barrier. The RH levels in the crawl space were higher than in the school building, and there was rust on the crawl space metal beams. In addition, the crawl space was under positive pressure, which allowed air from the crawl space to enter the school building, because the fan that generates the negative

Summary

(continued)

pressure (relative to the school) was not turned on. Samples taken from the new part of the school had lower fungal concentrations overall than those from the first floor of the renovated part. Significant concentrations of cat allergen were found on chairs in several classrooms and on the couch in the teachers' lounge. Recommendations to prevent water incursion and microbial growth are provided in this report.

Keywords: NAICS 611110 (Elementary and Secondary Schools), mold, ERMI, crawl space, cat allergen, dog allergen, IEQ, ventilation, visual contrast sensitivity, chronic biotoxin-related illness

On January 12, 2010, NIOSH received an employer request for an HHE at a middle school in Virginia because of staff concerns about exposure to mold in the school building. The requestor noted that more than a dozen employees had reported health complaints since the school underwent renovation in 2006–2007. A site visit was made on January 27–28, 2010. An opening conference was held with school administrators, county health department personnel, industrial hygiene consultants to the school district, and representatives from two teacher associations.

Building Description

The school has 137 staff and over 1000 students. A building engineer and seven custodians service the school. An informal system exists for reporting building issues to the engineer, who either deals with them personally or refers them to the Office of Facilities Management. Student health services at all schools in the district are provided by nurses from the county health department. The nurse that visits the school reported that student inhaler use and absenteeism were lower in this school than in other similar schools in the district. Employees receive health services through their private medical providers.

The school was built in the early 1960s. The two-story building was built mostly of concrete block and brick; we observed interior dry wall in one area of the school along Bevin Drive, near Room 122. The crawl space is shaped as a "T" and runs under the Bevan Drive and Main Street hallways. The facility has a flat roof. The original building was extensively renovated, and new administrative space, library, classrooms, VAV HVAC systems, electrical wiring, plumbing, and communications systems were added. The renovation and additions were completed by the start of the 2007–2008 school year.

Shortly after the renovation was completed, the teacher in Room 116 reported musty odors. An investigation revealed a connection between this room (behind a built-in cabinet) and the dirt-floored crawl space under the renovated part of the building. Moisture from the crawl space had led to microbial growth in the cabinet. This was repaired and the opening was sealed. No other significant microbial growth was identified by the school district. The school also identified some dry traps in the floor drains, which were emitting odors. These drains are now checked on a regular basis. A water pipe leaked in the

Introduction (continued)

band room practice area in the summer of 2009; the room was cleaned and the carpet dried before the start of the school year.

At the time of the HHE request, several staff members had seen a physician who conducts medical tests for mold illness. We were concerned that the mold tests performed by this physician were not in accordance with the generally accepted standard of medical practice. Some teachers had been on medical leave at the recommendation of this physician, reportedly due to illness from mold exposure. The presence of mold in the school was inferred from the results of four ERMI tests done by four staff members, with test results ranging from 1.06 to 6.93. (The ERMI scale ranges from about -10 to 20, the lowest to the highest. The closer the result is to 20, the greater the mold burden, indicating that there is likely to be significant water damage in that environment [Vesper et al. 2007].) The school district hired a consultant in 2009 to do a preliminary environmental assessment of the school and in 2010 to perform an industrial hygiene assessment of the building, focusing on IEQ and microbial growth.

Assessment

The employer provided an alphabetical list of the 137 employees, including teachers, custodians, cafeteria employees, administrative employees, counselors, and librarians. Research Randomizer (available at http://www.randomizer.com) was used to randomly generate a list of 72 employees for confidential medical interviews. In addition, the three employees who were on medical leave were contacted. Finally, an e-mail message was distributed by the principal's office to all employees to let them know they could be interviewed if they wanted to speak with us but were not on our list of randomly generated names. Medical records were requested if employees reported seeing a physician for health issues that they attributed to the school environment.

We observed workplace conditions, including the conditions in the crawl space. We reviewed the HVAC system balancing reports, current HVAC operations, and consultant reports and evaluated the effectiveness of the HVAC system. We measured pressure differentials between the classrooms and crawl space with a TSI Model 8705 DP-CALC® micromanometer (TSI Incorporated, Shoreview, Minnesota). A TRAMEX Moisture Encounter meter

(Tramex Ltd., Littleton, Colorado) was used to measure the interior wall moisture levels. Measurements of CO_2, CO, temperature, and RH were made throughout the work day with TSI Q-Trak™ Indoor Air Quality monitors (TSI Incorporated, Shoreview, Minnesota). The TSI Q-Trak monitors were pre- and post-calibrated at the NIOSH facility in Cincinnati, Ohio. Four samples were collected on sticky tape (SKC Inc., Eighty Four, Pennsylvania) from surfaces in the crawl space and gymnasium for microscopic fungal analysis. We also collected 10 dust samples from staff furniture to analyze for cat, dog, dust mite, and cockroach allergens, using a high-efficiency filter sock (Midwest Filtration Company, Fairfield, Ohio) with a HEPA vacuum. These samples were collected in areas where problems were reported and in areas not known to have problems. The dust samples were extracted with use of a phosphate-buffered saline solution and analyzed with an allergen ELISA screen at an AIHA-accredited laboratory.

Surfaces in 24 locations were wiped with a Swiffer® sheet (Procter & Gamble, Cincinnati, Ohio) and analyzed for the presence of fungal species by a DNA-based method called MSQPCR [Haugland et al. 2002]. The samples were collected from the top of the door frame; if not enough dust was present on the door frame, as many surfaces as possible, such as desks and bookcases, were dusted. In the analytical laboratory under a biosafety hood, the Swiffer sheets were opened and placed on a clean sheet of aluminum foil. The Swiffer sheets were vacuumed for 5 minutes with a Mi test sampler (Indoor Biotechnologies, Charlottesville, Virginia) attached to a Filter Queen Magestic vacuum cleaner (Health-Mor, Strongsville, Ohio). The dust was sieved and 5 milligrams of dust was weighed out for analysis with MSQPCR. MSQPCR identifies 36 species of fungi commonly associated with water-damaged indoor environments. Established procedures were used for preparing conidial suspensions from dust samples, extracting DNA, and performing MSQPCR analyses [Haugland et al. 2002; Brinkman et al. 2003; Haugland et al. 2004]. All primer and probe sequences, as well as known species composing the assay groups, were published at http://www.epa.gov/microbes/moldtech.htm. The ERMI is determined from the results of the analysis for 26 Group 1 mold species associated with water damage and 10 Group 2 or common species not associated with water damage [Meklin et al. 2004; Vesper et al. 2006]. The analysis of dust samples by MSQPCR from a national survey of homes conducted by HUD has produced the ERMI for United States homes [Vesper et al. 2007].

Sixty-eight employees were interviewed from the randomly generated list. The three employees on medical leave were interviewed, two over the telephone and one in person. Nine employees not on our list asked to be interviewed. Nineteen of the 80 (24%) interviewed employees were male. The average length of employment was 7 years (range: <1–24). Employees were asked about any medical problems or symptoms they had, and whether or not they thought the symptoms were related to the school environment.

Of the 68 randomly selected employees, 43 reported no symptoms related to the school environment. The most common reported symptoms related to the school environment were sinus infections or problems, eye irritation, muscle or joint aching or swelling, headaches, fatigue, and cough (Figure 1). Symptoms reported by less than five people included nasal symptoms such as runny or stuffy nose or irritation, sore or dry throat, memory problems, frequent upper respiratory infections, skin problems, dizziness, and shortness of breath. One employee reported being diagnosed with asthma in the past school year and that asthma symptoms were worse on days at work. Other medical issues reported by one employee each included peeling fingernails, change in hair texture, vitamin D deficiency, vocal cord nodules, Meniere's disease, racing heart, recurrent urinary frequency and urgency, tingling in various body parts, detached retina, and night sweats with fever and chills.

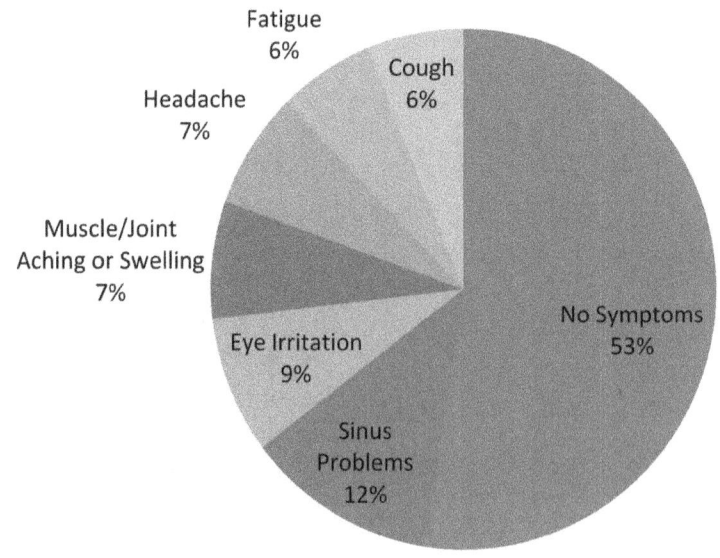

Figure 1. Symptoms Reported by Randomly Selected Employees (n=68).

Several employees reported that the physician who learned of the situation at the school after evaluating a few of the employees had set up a "clinic" to do an assessment of the middle school employees who wished to be evaluated by him. Most reported hearing about this clinic from their co-workers. The employees who participated in this private clinic were asked if they experienced a long list of symptoms, including fatigue, weakness, headache, red eyes, tearing, sinus, cough, diarrhea, joint pain, memory problems, mood swings, appetite change, metallic tastes, and tremor. They had blood drawn for numerous tests* and had VCS testing by the physician. No medical history or physical exam or informed consent was obtained. Each employee later received a letter that contained their lab results, along with a "master list" of test results and symptoms for all 22 employees from the school that were screened, with names removed. The participants were not provided with an individual interpretation of their results, but the letter instructed the participants to determine if they are a "case" by comparing their results to a specified list of test results and symptoms that was included in the letter. The employees were then told to contact their personal physicians and to request a new-patient packet if they wanted to be seen in his office after consulting with their personal physician.

In addition, several of the laboratory reports of "clinic" tests included the following statements:

- "This test uses a kit/reagent designated by the manufacturer as for research use, not for clinical use.... It has not been cleared or approved by the U.S. Food and Drug Administration. The results are not intended to be used as the sole means for clinical diagnosis or patient management decisions...."

- "[This test] is an investigational assay. Clinical application has not been fully defined."

- "For research use only."

Of the 12 employees who either requested NIOSH interviews or were interviewed on medical leave, 2 reported no symptoms related to the school environment. The most commonly reported

---

*Human leukocyte antigens class 1 and 2, vasoactive intestinal polypeptide, melanocyte stimulating hormone, leptin, antidiuretic hormone, osmolality, adrenocorticotropic hormone, cortisol, dehydroepiandrosterone sulfate, testosterone, androstenedione, transforming growth factor beta 1, plasminogen activator inhibitor 1, vascular endothelial growth factor, C3a, C4a, immunoglobulin E, Lyme Western blot, thyroid stimulating hormone, anticardiolipin antibodies, tissue transglutaminase IgA, antigliadin IgG and IgA, ferritin, and Von Willebrand factor.

symptoms were sinus infections or problems and muscle or joint aching or swelling (4 people each); eye irritation, memory problems, nausea, and insomnia (3 each); headaches, fatigue, and dizziness (2 each); and nasal symptoms such as runny or stuffy nose or irritation, sore or dry throat, skin problems, wheezing, and shortness of breath (1 each). One employee had been seen by multiple physicians and evaluated for multiple sclerosis, lupus, and rheumatoid arthritis. This employee was being treated by a physician for "chronic neurotoxin disease." One reported being diagnosed with "biotoxin mediated illness." Another employee reported developing Lyme disease after a tick bite, with resulting joint pain and swelling. The employee felt the Lyme disease was exacerbated by the school environment. Another employee reported getting a severe headache that persisted for several days after a colonoscopy and felt this was related to the school environment. The last three employees reported being treated with cholestyramine, and one reported being treated with erythropoietin for these symptoms.

Because the ERMI values calculated from the dust samples that we collected were higher in the renovated part of the school than in the new part, the percentage of employees reporting symptoms they related to the school environment was calculated according to building location. Fifty percent (20/40) of employees interviewed whose primary location was the first floor of the renovated part reported symptoms, as did 48% (13/27) of employees whose primary location was in the new part, 20% (1/5) of employees who worked on the second floor of the renovated part, and 29% (2/7) who worked throughout the building.

Medical records were reviewed for seven employees, two of whom had seen more than one physician. Medical records for 15 employees who reported having seen the physician who had conducted the "clinic" were repeatedly requested from the physician, but these were never received. Records were reviewed for an employee who had recently been diagnosed with asthma. It appeared that the diagnosis was based upon spirometry that did not meet acceptability and reproducibility criteria set forth by the American Thoracic Society. Also, the pattern on spirometry was predominantly restrictive, which is not an indication of airway obstruction (the pattern seen in asthma). None of the other records documented a work-related medical problem.

Environmental Assessment

HVAC Systems

The VAV HVAC system has five zones served by separate air-handling units (Zones A–E), with perimeter heating units in the entrances. We inspected two rooftop air-handling units (E1 and A2). These units were clean, the drain pans were dry, and the pleated filters fit well. The pleated filters (Purolator Defiant Mack 80-D™) were classified as MERV 8 (which meets the ANSI/ASHRAE recommendation of MERV 6 or higher) and are changed quarterly. The balance reports showed that all of the HVAC units had been tested before the reopening of the school after renovation. There was no information concerning balancing after reoccupancy.

The occupied mode was from 6:30 a.m. to 11:30 p.m., which provided heating or cooling depending upon the season when the thermostat setting was reached. The occupied set point temperatures ranged from 69°F to 74°F. The regular classroom VAV HVAC units were on a partial recirculating system that used a common open ceiling plenum and, according to management, provided a minimum of 20% outdoor air. The science classrooms had dedicated single-pass HVAC systems. An ozone-generating air cleaner was observed in Room 122. Ozone generators have been identified as a source of health problems in the indoor environment [U.S. EPA 2010], and a current policy at the school prohibits their use.

Indoor Environmental Quality Parameters

In January 2010, IEQ parameters (CO_2, CO, temperature, and RH) were continually measured in 5 classrooms with VAV HVAC systems over a 23-hour period (Table 1). Figures A1–A5 in Appendix A show the IEQ parameter data in graphic form. The classrooms were occupied during the day. Rooms 102, 116, 122, and 136 were in the renovated part of the school, and Room 202 was in the new part of the school. Spot checks for IEQ parameters were also made outdoors for comparison and in the crawl space (Table 1). We found CO_2 concentrations in the four classrooms in the renovated part of the building ranged up to 2648 ppm, which exceeded recommended ANSI/ASHRAE guidelines [ANSI/ASHRAE 2010a]. The windows in Room 136 were open during the sampling period, and low levels of CO (range: 0 ppm to 0.8 ppm) were detected; these were below levels measured outside.

Nearby automobile traffic is the likely source of the CO detected. The temperatures and RH levels in the classrooms were within expected ranges for the heating season [ANSI/ASHRAE 2010b]. Spot check measurements in the crawl space showed that the RH levels were higher in the crawl space than in the occupied area. Additional information concerning the ANSI/ASHRAE guidelines can be found in Appendix B.

Table 1. Measurements of IEQ parameters (CO_2, CO, temperature, and RH)

Sample Location	Carbon Dioxide Range (ppm)	Carbon Monoxide Range (ppm)	Temperature Range (°F)	Relative Humidity Range (%)
Continuous Measurements				
Room 102	406–1371	0	71.6–76.1	16.4–24.8
Room 116	399–1591	0	68–73	17.9–26.5
Room 122	415–1229	0	66.6–72.3	16.1–22.6
Room 136	405–2648	0–0.8	66–77.2	14.9–33.3
Room 202	322–921	0	69.4–73.8	14.5–20.3
Spot Checks				
Outdoors	458–509	0–3.1	43.7–45	24.3–26.3
Crawl Space	600–900	0	60	61–67

Observations and Airflow Measurements

In the main gymnasium, there was an accumulation of material along the seams of the sound panels. The sticky-tape samples showed that it was mostly dust with a few mold spores (Table 2). It was reported to us that school district facility employees removed the sound panels and found open expansion joints in the exterior walls. These were caulked and the sound panels were cleaned and reinstalled after our site visit.

We found three small isolated areas of visible mold growth during our evaluation. Two were cardboard boxes (one in the crawl space next to the boiler room [Figure 2] and one in the laundry room drain) and one was on a wall next to a leaking pipe in the teachers' lounge, next to Room 122. Dr. Vesper, from U.S. EPA, analyzed a tape sample from the laundry room box and identified the main fungi as *Stachybotrys* spp. *Stachybotrys* is found in soil and prefers to grow on decaying plant material, cellulose, and wallboard under wet conditions. Tape samples from the cardboard box in the crawl space showed the presence of *Acremonium* and *Dicyma* organisms (Table 2). Both *Acremonium* and *Dicyma* require wet conditions to grow. *Acremonium* is found in soil and *Dicyma* prefers to grow on dead plants, paper, and cardboard.

Table 2. Results of microscopic analysis of sticky-tape samples

Location	Genera	Spores/cm²
Dust from gym acoustic panel	Cladosporium	0.21
	Epicoccum	0.21
	Smuts, Periconia, Myxomycetes	0.21
Dust from gym acoustic panel	Smuts, Periconia, Myxomycetes	0.21
Cardboard in crawl space	Acremonium	0.21
	Dicyma	70,000
Cardboard in crawl space	Acremonium	140,000
	Dicyma	74,000

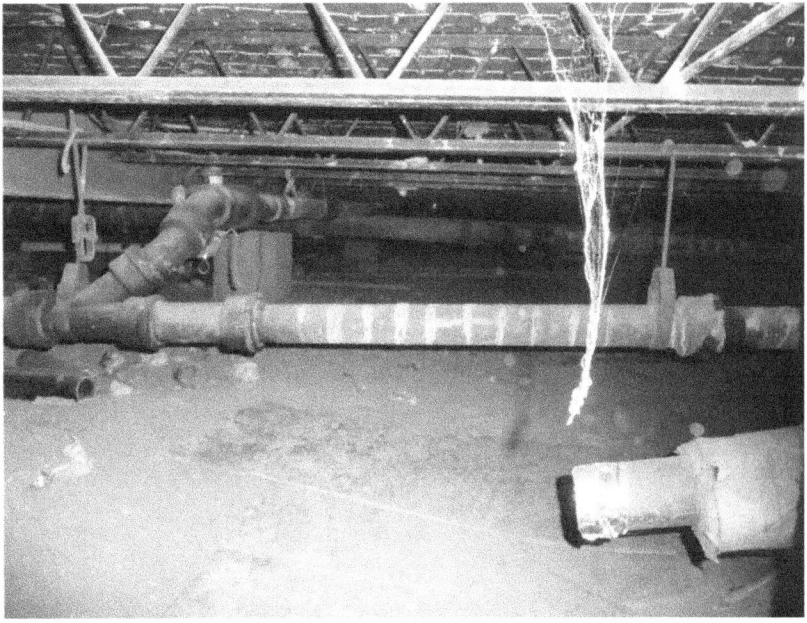

Figure 2. Crawl space next to the boiler room, showing rusty pipes and a moldy cardboard box (on the floor) that was removed during our visit.

We entered the crawl space through Room 007N and visually inspected a small portion of the crawl space area. The air in the crawl space under the renovated part of the building was more humid than the outside air. The crawl space was positive to the room (+0.0001 to 0.0025" water) at the time of the site visit, which means that air was flowing into the room from the crawl space. The room was also positive to the hallway (+0.01" water), which means that air was flowing from the room into the hallway. The exhaust fan for the crawl space was rated at 1215 CFM (tested March 17, 2008, at 1292 CFM). Air gaps around the pipes allow air to enter the building from the crawl space. Some areas of the crawl space have a plastic moisture barrier. There was no standing water in the portion of the crawl space that we entered. In several areas along the perimeter of the building and in the courtyard, the grading surrounding the building is sloped toward the building and could result in additional moisture in the crawl space and school (Figure 3). We checked the moisture levels in walls for the teachers' lounge, adjacent to Room 122; in Storage Room 7A; and the wall across from Room 122 and found that all measurements were within acceptable ranges.

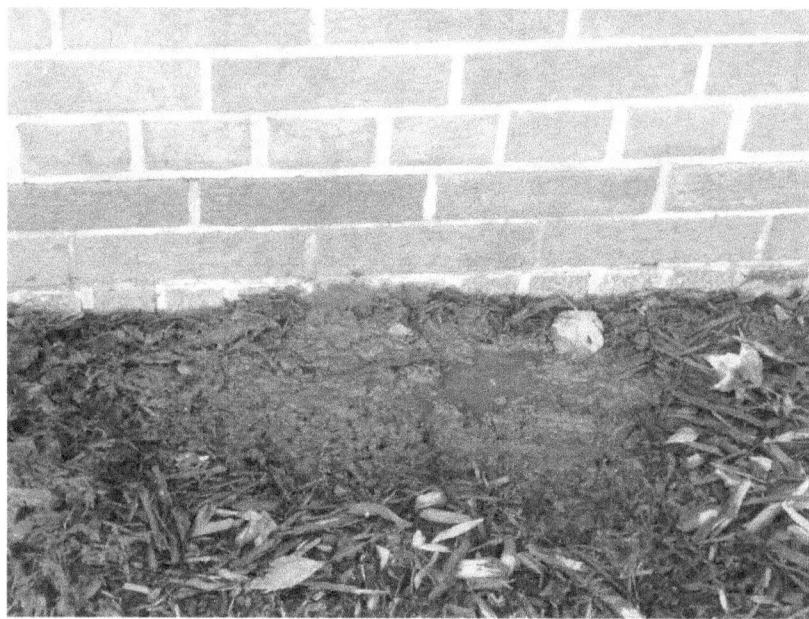

Figure 3. Water pooling at the edge of a wall inside the courtyard.

In some areas, we found stained or wet ceiling tiles (Room 7A and the hallway outside of the teachers' lounge, by Room 116) but no obvious signs of microbial growth on these ceiling tiles. Rainwater had entered the school in the hallway outside Room 16 through one of the rooftop HVAC units the week prior to the site visit. The storm had come from a different direction than usual, and the HVAC unit was not protected by metal barriers. School management reported to us that, since our site visit, they have identified and repaired the roof leaks and barrier issues that resulted in the water damage.

There has been an ongoing sewage backup problem in the women's locker room in the new gymnasium, which also backs up into the physical education teacher's shower area. The school maintenance staff suspects that the low-flow toilets installed during the renovation cannot handle disposal of feminine hygiene products. They have used a plumbing snake to remove the blockages.

Allergens

The levels of cat, dog, dust mite, and cockroach allergens in samples collected from the chairs and couch in the classrooms, offices, and teachers' lounge are listed in Table A1 in Appendix A. We found that six of the ten dust samples had levels in the range of 1–8 µg/g of cat allergen (Fel d1), a range that has been associated with sensitization of humans [Liccardi et al. 2003]. The other four samples had detectable, though lower, levels of cat allergen. All ten samples had detectable levels of dog allergen (Can f1), nine of which were in the 1–2 µg/g range that has been associated with sensitization [AIHA 2005]. Two samples were positive for dust mite allergen (one each for Der f1 and Der p1), but the concentrations were below the 2-µg/g level associated with sensitization [AIHA 2005]. No cockroach allergen was detected in these samples at the laboratory limit of detection.

Environmental Relative Moldiness Index (ERMI)

Table 3 shows the ERMI values for each of the sampled rooms. The complete ERMI data for each room are found in Appendix A, Table A2. The ERMI tests from January 2010 showed that Rooms 116, 120, 122, 127, 130, 131, and 136, above the crawl space, had higher ERMI values (1.82 to 9.65) than areas in the new part of the school. A wide diversity of fungal species was identified. In general, Rooms 210, 211, 213, and 217 on the second floor of the renovated part of the school had lower ERMI values (3.31 to 5.66) than those rooms above the crawl space. Classrooms 142 and 143, around the courtyard, had ERMI values ranging from -0.35 to 6.10. The samples collected in the new part of the school (Rooms 100A, 101, 102, 105, 106, 107) had very low ERMI values (-2.38 to 3.2), and the one sample from the office area (002B) was -0.76. Several of these samples (Rooms 002B, 101, 102, 105, 106 and 122) had low sample weights, indicating that the rooms were clean and there was little dust to collect. The two boiler rooms had ERMI values of 0.10 and 6.74. The storage closet in Room 143 had the highest value (18.63). Management reported that this room was not cleaned after a moldy cloth had been removed in the fall of 2009 and the exhaust fan was not working. The room has since been cleaned and the fan repaired.

Table 3. Summary of ERMI values

Room Number	ERMI
002B*	-0.76
100A	3.2
101*	-2.38
102*	-1.97
105*	-1.73
106*	2.86
107	-0.76
116NS	9.65
120	1.82
122*	2.57
122NS	6.08
127NS	6.02
130NS	9.27
Boiler	6.74
Boiler	6.10
131NS	9.07
136	0.78
142	-1.35
143	6.10
143NS	18.63
210NS	5.66
211NS	6.44
213NS	3.31
217NS	3.72

*low sample weight
NS – nonstandard – dust collected around room

Consultant Reports

We reviewed the following information: a March 2010 report from a consulting company hired by the school district, and a series of expert witness letter reports provided by a private attorney to the school district, dated September 2010. These reports are summarized below.

The consulting company conducted several evaluations at the school from November 2009 until February 2010. The consulting company evaluated moisture content in the school, using infrared thermal imaging, and conducted visual inspections throughout the school building, crawl space, HVAC units, and VAV boxes for the areas over Bevan Drive. They found the building and HVAC units to be well-maintained. They did find grading issues outside near Room 07B, which resulted in excess moisture in that area. They did not find any visible mold growth in the building, but they identified at least 40 stained ceiling tiles during their inspections. They reported that the ductwork for Room 116 had a higher particulate load than the other inspected ductwork, but they did not find visible mold growth in the ductwork or VAV boxes. Standing water was observed in the crawl space in December 2009. The consulting company also found that the crawl space was under either neutral or positive pressure with respect to the school building. They conducted a formal survey of the school staff to determine IEQ issues and investigated the reported issues, mostly related to odors. Air, surface-wipe, and sticky-tape samples were collected for mold analysis, and a limited number of air samples were collected for bacterial analysis. The concentrations of mold were lower inside than outside for culturable and spore trap samples. The genera of detected mold indoors were similar to those in outdoor samples. They noted that snow cover outside likely kept outside mold concentrations low. The wipe sample from the acoustic panels in the gymnasium did not show mold growth. The air samples taken from the crawl space and analyzed for *Actinomycetes* (bacteria) showed no growth.

In June 2010, expert witnesses hired by an attorney evaluated the construction and building design and the HVAC systems and collected air, dust, and sticky-tape samples for mold, focusing on "complaint" areas. They reported a wide range of issues with ventilation in the crawl space; high humidity levels; unsealed penetrations from the crawl space and roof; visible mold contamination on tar paper and pipe insulation in the crawl space; missing roof flashing, leading to leakage in the building; lack of HVAC system balancing and proper operation; mold growth, plant material, and pollen grains on the VAV boxes and air ducts for Rooms 115, 116, and 122; and the presence of mold spores associated with damp environments (*Chaetomium* and *Stachybotrys*) in air and dust samples collected in the crawl space, Room 116, Room 120, Room 007B, and the library.

Discussion

Many buildings have episodes of water or moisture incursion. Mold comprises 25% of the biomass of the earth; therefore, mold will always be present in the soil. The key to preventing mold growth is to identify the source of moisture and to eliminate it. Although the ERMI was developed to evaluate homes rather than to determine whether or not a school or commercial building has evidence of fungal contamination, we can compare the ERMI results from one part of the building to another. Samples taken from the new part of the school had lower ERMI values overall than those from the first floor of the renovated part. The prevalence of symptoms or illness related to the school environment by employees, however, did not differ by area. The crawl space under the renovated part of the building has a dirt floor with a partial moisture barrier, and the soil ouside the building sloped toward the foundation instead of away from it, allowing water to enter the crawl space.

At the time of our visit in January 2010, there was no visible mold growth or standing water in the crawl space but there was moisture under the partial moisture barrier. The RH readings in the crawl space were higher than in the school building, and there was rust on the crawl space metal beams. In addition, the crawl space was under positive pressure because the fan that generates negative pressure relative to the school was not turned on. There are also pipe perforations through the floor, which allow air movement between the crawl space and the renovated part of the school. The most likely explanation for the higher ERMI values in the renovated part of the school is moisture incursion from the crawl space. In addition, some rooms with VAV HVAC units had high CO_2 concentrations, which may indicate insufficient introduction of outdoor air.

We found significant concentrations of cat allergen on the chairs in several classrooms and the couch in the teachers' lounge. Allergies to cat and dog dander, dust mites, and cockroaches have been linked to asthma exacerbation [IOM 2000; Macher et al. 2005]. Upholstered furniture that is not frequently cleaned is a significant allergen reservoir [Tranter et al. 2009]. A detailed discussion of IEQ issues, including mold, is in Appendix B.

Our environmental findings suggest that mold incursion is occurring through connections between the crawl space and the occupied space in the renovated part of the building, but the patterns and rates of symptoms do not suggest a relationship to the school environment. In our medical interviews, randomly selected employees reported common symptoms similar to those reported in a large study of buildings without IEQ complaints and in the general population.

There was heightened awareness of the suspected mold problem in the school; employees reported being urged to get tested at the private physician's "clinic" that was set up specifically for school employees. Such heightened awareness might lead individuals to notice symptoms they might otherwise overlook and to attribute them to the work environment. Care must be taken when attributing common symptoms to particular exposures, because the association is as likely to be coincidental as to be causal. A symptom is any subjective sensation or perceived change in bodily function, such as low-back pain and fatigue, which only the individual can perceive. In contrast, a sign is objective evidence of disease that is evident to the health care provider, such as a bloody nose or a red eye. Symptoms are influenced by cognitive (thought) processes [Bogaerts et al. 2010]. Symptoms have been demonstrated to be more common when pollution or health threats are perceived, as at this school [Watson and Pennebaker 1989; Williams and Lees-Haley 1993], and can be affected by fears, emotional triggers, and litigation [Lees-Haley and Brown 1992].

Of the general population, 86%–95% have one or more common symptoms during any given 2- to 4-week period, and the average adult reports a minimum of one symptom every 4 to 6 days [Barsky and Borus 1995]. These symptoms are rarely caused by serious illness. In fact, 15%–50% of primary care visits are for what is termed "medically unexplained symptoms" [Kroenke 2001; Kirmayer et al. 2004; Jackson et al. 2009; Bogaerts et al. 2010]. Medically unexplained symptoms are those for which no cause is found, even after thorough medical evaluation. Lipscomb et al. reported 1-year symptom prevalence rates from three populations in California [Lipscomb et al. 1992]. The top 10 symptoms were sinus congestion or sneeze, irritated eyes, allergies or asthma, headaches, fatigue, difficulty sleeping, numbness or tingling in limbs, and skin problems, with rates ranging from 9.1% to 30.4%. A similar study in Australia found the top 10 symptoms were stuffy nose, headaches, fatigue, cough, itchy eyes, sore throat, skin rash, wheezing, trouble breathing, and nausea, with rates ranging from 10.1% to 46.2% [Heyworth and McCaul 2001]. The U.S. EPA conducted a systematic survey of 100 randomly selected office buildings without known IEQ complaints in the United States to develop baseline data about U.S. office buildings [Brightman et al. 2008]. NIOSH conducted a similar study of 80 buildings with IEQ complaints [Malkin et al. 1996]. Occupants in both studies reported work-related symptoms. The rank order of symptoms was the same, but rates were significantly higher in the buildings with IEQ complaints. The most common work-related symptoms reported in both studies were dry, itching, or irritated eyes; unusual tiredness or fatigue; headache; tension or irritability; pain in back, neck, and shoulders; stuffy or runny nose, or sinus congestion; sneezing; sore or dry throat; and difficulty remembering things or concentrating. Forty-five percent of the employees in the randomly selected buildings reported at least one work-related symptom. These common symptoms in the general population and in buildings are also the most common symptoms reported by school employees.

The average adult has two to three upper respiratory infections per year [Benninger et al. 2003]. Sinusitis is the most frequently reported chronic disease in the United States, topping arthritis, allergies, and hypertension [Benson and Marano 1993]. Thirteen percent of U.S. adults reported physician-diagnosed sinusitis in 2008, according to the National Health Interview Survey [CDC 2009].

Several employees reported specific medical diagnoses that are unrelated to each other and to the school environment, for example, Lyme disease, Meniere's disease, and vitamin D deficiency. Others had symptoms potentially suggestive of diagnosable medical conditions, such as change in hair texture, recurrent urinary frequency and urgency, and night sweats with fever and chills. It is important that employees seek appropriate medical care; such care could include a proper medical evaluation concerning work-relatedness of symptoms. Inappropriate attribution of these symptoms to the workplace can lead to delays in diagnosis and treatment or to harm from inappropriate treatment.

DISCUSSION
(CONTINUED)

The use of questionnaires to determine patient symptoms in the clinical setting has been repeatedly demonstrated to be prone to overendorsement of symptoms, which means they consistently result in a greater number of symptoms being reported than patients would have reported on their own, sometimes up to four times more [Homsi et al. 2006; Nolin et al. 2006; Stapleton and Mills 2008; Iverson et al. 2010]. Thus, the use of a list of over 30 nonspecific symptoms by the private physician who set up the "clinic" likely led to more people being labeled as ill or as a "case" than would have been without the use of the list.

Two published studies claim that biotoxin-related illness is a condition with multiple-organ-system symptoms related to water-damaged buildings [Shoemaker and House 2005; Shoemaker and House 2006]. Both studies used VCS to document and monitor the illness. Interpretation of these studies is hampered by methodological limitations, including a nonrepresentative sample, medical conditions that often present with multisystem symptoms (e.g., fibromyalgia and chronic fatigue syndrome), the lack of a comparison group, and poor exposure characterization. Replication of findings by other researchers is a critical element in confirming hypotheses such as this. NIOSH investigators have used VCS testing in an investigation to see if it could be used as a marker of effect from occupancy in water-damaged buildings. We concluded that VCS should not be used for clinical assessment of individuals exposed to water-damaged buildings [NIOSH 2010].

Many of the blood tests that school employees underwent for the private physician are not approved by the Food and Drug Administration, are for research purposes only, or were interpreted in a nonstandard manner. The laboratory reports that we reviewed also contained claims of validity and certification. Validity of a test's performance characteristics means that the test measures what it says it will measure and that the laboratory methods give accurate, precise, and reliable results. While a test may be valid for measuring a particular substance, measurement of that substance may not be appropriate in the diagnosis or treatment of a specific illness. Laboratories, not tests, are certified under the Clinical Laboratory Improvement Amendments of 1988 (CLIA-88). Having a test performed in a CLIA-certified laboratory does not mean that the clinician used the test results appropriately for diagnosis.

While it is critical to pursue research to expand our knowledge base, it is also critical to present research or experimental

Discussion
(continued)

diagnostic procedures as such, with the full informed consent of each participant. While cholestyramine is unlikely to cause significant harm, all medications are approved for specific uses and all have potential side effects; therefore all medication use should be evaluated carefully. In addition, some medications, including erythropoietin, have risks determined by the Food and Drug Administration to be worthy of extra warnings, such as a black box warning [FDA 2009]. A black box warning is designed to call attention to serious or life-threatening risks of certain prescription drugs. We have serious concerns about employees being given this potentially harmful medication in a different way than described in the Food and Drug Administration approved drug label.

Conclusions

We identified several correctable structural problems at the school. The main issue was that the crawl space under the renovated part of the school was a potential source of mold and dampness because of improper grading of the soil and inadequate ventilation. The high CO_2 concentrations indicated that, at times, the VAV HVAC system was not supplying enough outdoor air. Cat and dog allergen levels were elevated on some of the furniture that was sampled and could have contributed to work-related allergy symptoms of employees who have cat or dog allergies.

Many of the symptoms reported by employees, such as sinus problems and headaches, are common in offices, schools, and the general population. There is no evidence that more serious health problems reported by some staff are related to working in the building. These illnesses require medical diagnosis and treatment based on generally recognized and accepted medical practice, with the understanding that not all symptoms have a simple explanation. The lack of a ready explanation for all symptoms has led some employees to seek nonstandard medical care.

On the basis of our findings, we recommend the actions listed below to create a more healthful workplace. We encourage the school to use a labor-management health and safety committee or working group to discuss the recommendations in this report and develop an action plan. Those involved in the work can best set priorities and assess the feasibility of our recommendations for the specific situation at the school. Our recommendations are based on the hierarchy of controls approach. This approach groups actions by their likely effectiveness in reducing or removing hazards. In most cases, the preferred approach is to eliminate hazardous materials or processes and install engineering controls to reduce exposure or shield employees. Until such controls are in place, or if they are not effective or feasible, administrative measures and/or personal protective equipment may be needed.

Engineering Controls

Engineering controls reduce exposures to employees by removing the hazard from the process or placing a barrier between the hazard and the employee. Engineering controls are very effective at protecting employees without placing primary responsibility of implementation on the employee.

1. Address the movement of potentially contaminated air from the crawl space into the school building. This can be accomplished by maintaining negative pressure in the crawl space, adding a moisture barrier, and sealing the floor penetrations [IICRC 2006].

2. Test and balance the VAV boxes to ensure adequate ventilation to all occupied areas. ANSI/ASHRSE recommends an outdoor air supply rate of 10 CFM/person for classrooms. Use the highest-efficiency filters that the HVAC system can handle to reduce the potential for mold spores to enter the HVAC system. Do not use windows in the classrooms to reduce the entrance of unfiltered, unconditioned air.

3. Identify and fix indoor roof water leaks in a timely matter.

4. Regrade the soil around the building to ensure water does not collect at the foundation and in the crawl space.

5. Remove all porous items (such as carpeting and carpet padding, upholstery, wallpaper, ceiling tiles, paper, books, etc.) that have been wet for more than 48 hours and that cannot be thoroughly cleaned and dried. These items can remain a source of mold growth and should be removed from the school.

RECOMMENDATIONS (CONTINUED)

Administrative Controls

Administrative controls are management-dictated work practices and policies to reduce or prevent exposures to workplace hazards. The effectiveness of administrative changes in work practices for controlling workplace hazards is dependent on management commitment and employee acceptance. Regular monitoring and reinforcement is necessary to ensure that control policies and procedures are not circumvented in the name of convenience or production.

1. Institute a training program concerning the proper disposal of feminine hygiene products to address the plumbing issue in the women's gymnasium locker room toilets.

2. Vacuum the furniture in the school with a HEPA vacuum on a regular basis to remove allergens.

3. Implement an IEQ management plan for the school district. An IEQ manager or administrator with clearly defined responsibilities, authority, and resources should be selected. This individual should have a good understanding of the building's structure and function and should be able to effectively communicate with occupants. This is a proactive approach that can help prevent IEQ problems from occurring. Although comprehensive regulatory standards specific to IEQ have not been established, guidelines have been developed by organizations such as ASHRAE, NIOSH, and the U.S. EPA. The U.S. EPA has several publications on IEQ, including the *IAQ Tools for Schools Action Kit* which is available at http://www.epa.gov/iaq/schools/toolkit.html. The *Tools for Schools* document discusses IEQ in some detail and includes information on common problems, investigative techniques, and solutions to specific problems. Additional resources include the U.S. EPA Healthy School Environments Assessment Tool, available at http://www.epa.gov/schools/, which helps school districts establish and manage comprehensive school facility self-assessment programs. It contains an environmental health and safety checklist and is designed to be easily customized to reflect state and local requirements and policies. The basic elements of a good IEQ plan include the following:

- Properly operating and maintaining HVAC equipment, including accommodating occupants who work during hours when the HVAC system is routinely cycled off, to ensure that adequate ventilation is provided.

- Overseeing the activities of occupants and contractors that affect IEQ (e.g., housekeeping, pest control, maintenance, food preparation).

- Maintaining and ensuring effective and timely communication with occupants regarding IEQ.

- Educating building occupants and contractors about their responsibilities in relation to IEQ.

- Proactively identifying and managing projects that may affect IEQ (e.g , redecoration, renovation, relocation of personnel).

- Designating a school employee representative who can speak for the teachers and other employees and can assist with communication.

Information on selecting IEQ consultants, if needed, is available from the AIHA *Guidelines for Selecting an Indoor Air Quality Consultant.*

4. Encourage employees with health concerns to seek evaluation and care from a physician who is residency trained and board certified in occupational medicine and is familiar with the types of exposures employees may have had and their health effects. You can locate these occupational medicine physicians through a variety of sources, including the Association of Occupational and Environmental Clinics, at http://www.aoec.org, and the American College of Occupational and Environmental Medicine, at http://www.acoem.org. The University of Maryland has a large occupational and environmental medicine clinic that could serve all your needs. It may be useful to provide the physician with a copy of this report.

5. Work with employee associations to inform employees about the limitations and potential risks of nonstandard medical tests and treatments. Refrain from participating in nonstandard medical testing and treatments without full knowledge and informed consent of risks and benefits. Consultation with staff from a university occupational and environmental medicine clinic is recommended.

6. Implement a formal system for reporting building concerns to the building manager. This system can be paper or electronic and should include a mechanism for the building manager to let staff know when and how the problem is fixed.

RECOMMENDATIONS (CONTINUED)

The following is a general recommendation that will improve IEQ in any facility and is not based upon specific problems we identified at the school.

7. Appoint an individual or group to research and approve cleaning materials used in your school district. Because there are no regulations regarding what can be labeled "environmentally friendly," this individual or group will need to become knowledgeable about what cleaning materials are appropriate. Useful sources of information to help select the safest products include the National Institutes of Health database [http://householdproducts.nlm.nih.gov/], the Greenguard Environmental Institute [http://www.greenguard.org], Green Seal [http://www.greenseal.org/], and Terra Choice [http://www.terrachoice.com/]. The Healthy School Network [http://www.healthyschools.org/] has examples of other school districts that have revamped their housekeeping and maintenance programs.

REFERENCES

AIHA [2005]. Chapter 8: Indoor allergens. In: Field guide for the determination of biological contaminant in environmental samples. Hung LL, Miller JD, Dillon KH, eds. Fairfax, VA: American Industrial Hygiene Association.

ANSI/ASHRAE [2010a]. Ventilation for acceptable indoor air quality. American National Standards Institute/ASHRAE standard 62.1-2010. Atlanta, GA: American Society of Heating, Refrigerating, and Air-Conditioning Engineers, Inc.

ANSI/ASHRAE [2010b]. Thermal environmental conditions for human occupancy. American National Standards Institute/ASHRAE standard 55-2010. Atlanta, GA: American Society for Heating, Refrigerating, and Air-Conditioning Engineers, Inc.

Barsky AJ, Borus JF [1995]. Somatization and medicalization in the era of managed care. JAMA 274(24):1931-1934.

Benninger MS, Ferguson BJ, Hadley JA, Hamilos DL, Jacobs M, Kennedy DW, Lanza DC, Marple BF, Osguthorpe JD, Stankiewicz JA, Anon J, Denneny J, Emanuel I, Levine H [2003]. Adult chronic rhinosinusitis: definitions, diagnosis, epidemiology, and pathophysiology. Otolayngol Head Neck Surg 129(3 Suppl):S1-S32.

Benson V, Marano MA [1993]. Current estimates from the National Health Interview Survey, 1993, National Center for Health Statistics. Vital Health Stat 10(182).

Bogaerts K, Van Eylen L, Li W, Bresseleers J, Van Diest I, De Peuter S, Stans L, Decramer M, Van den Bergh O [2010]. Distorted symptom perception in patients with medically unexplained symptoms. J Abnorm Pschyol 119(1):226-234.

Brightman HS, Milton DK, Wypij D, Burge HA, Spengler JD [2008]. Evaluating building-related symptoms using the US EPA BASE study results. Indoor Air 18(4):335-345.

Brinkman NE, Haugland RA, Wymer LJ, Byappanahalli M, Whitman RL, Vesper SJ [2003]. Evaluation of a rapid, quantitative real-time PCR method for cellular enumeration of pathogenic Candida species in water. Appl Environ Microbiol 69(3):1775-1782.

CDC [2009]. Summary Health Statistics for U.S. Adults: National Health Interview Survey,2008. available at http://www.cdc.gov/nchs/nhis/nhis_series.htm. Date accessed: March 2011.

FDA [2009]. Public Health Advisory: erythropoiesis-stimulating agents (ESAs). Available at http://www.fda.gov/ForConsumers/ByAudience/ForPatientAdvocates/HIVandAIDSActivities/ucm124262.htm. Date accessed: March 2011.

Haugland RA, Brinkman NE, Vesper SJ [2002]. Evaluation of rapid DNA extraction methods for the quantitative detection of fungal cells using real time PCR analysis. J Microbiol Meth 50(3):319-323.

Haugland RA, Varma M, Wymer LJ, Vesper SJ [2004]. Quantitative PCR of selected Aspergillus, Penicillium and Paecilomyces species. Sys Appl Microbiol 27(2):198-210.

Heyworth J, McCaul K [2001]. Prevalence of non-specific health symptoms in South Australia. Int J Environ Health Res 11(4):291-298.

Homsi J, Walsh D, Rivera N, Rybicki LA, Nelson KA, Legrand SB, Davis M, Naughton M, Gvozdjan D, Pham H [2006]. Symptom evaluation in palliative medicine: patient report vs. systematic assessment. Support Care Cancer 14(5):444-453.

IICRC [2006]. Standard and reference guide for professional water damage restoration, IICRC 500. Vancouver, Washington: Institute of Inspection, Cleaning, and Restoration. ANSI/IICRC S500-2006.

IOM [2000]. Executive Summary. In: Clearing the air: asthma and indoor air exposure. Institute of Medicine, National Academy Press, Washington, DC. pp. 1–18.

Iverson GL, Brooks BL, Ashton VL, Lange RT [2010]. Interview versus questionnaire symptom reporting in people with the postconcussion syndrome. J Head Trauma Rehab 25(1):23–30.

Jackson JL, George S, Hinchey S [2009]. Medically unexplained physical symptoms. J Gen Intern Med 24(4):540–542.

Kirmayer LJ, Groleau D, Looper KJ, Dominice Dao M [2004]. Explaining medically unexplained symptoms. Can J Psychiatry 49(10):663–672.

Kroenke K [2001]. Studying symptoms: sampling and measurement issues. Ann Intern Med 134(9 part 2):844–853.

Lees-Haley PR, Brown RS [1992]. Bias in perception and reporting following a perceived toxic exposure. Percept Mot Skills 75(2):531–544.

Liccardi G, D'Amato G, Russo M, Canonica GW, D'Amato L, De Martino M, Passalacqua G [2003]. Focus on cat allergen (Fel d 1): immunological and aerodynamic characteristics, modality of airway sensitization and avoidance strategies. Int Arch Allergy Immunol 132(1):1–12.

Lipscomb JA, Satin KP, Neutra RR [1992]. Reported symptom prevalence rates from comparison populations in community-based environmental studies. Arch Environ Health 47(4)263–269.

Macher JM, Tsai FC, Burton LE, Liu KS [2005]. Concentrations of cat and dust-mite allergens in dust samples from 92 large US office buildings from the BASE Study. Indoor Air 15(Suppl 9):82–88.

Malkin R, Wicox T, Sieber WK [1996]. The National Institute for Occupational Safety and Health indoor environmental evaluation experience. Part two: symptom prevalence. Appl Occup Environ Hyg 11(6):540–545.

Meklin T, Haugland RA, Reponen T, Varma M, Lummus Z, Bernstein D, Wymer LJ, Vesper SJ [2004]. Quantitative PCR analysis of house dust can reveal abnormal mold conditions. J Environ Monit 6(7):615-20.

NIOSH [2010]. Health hazard evaluation report: comparison of mold exposures, work-related symptoms, and visual contrast sensitivity between employees at a severely water-damaged school and employees at a school without significant water damage, New Orleans, LA. By Thomas G, Burton NC, Mueller C, Page E. Cincinnati, OH: U.S. Department of Health and Human Services, Centers for Disease Control and Prevention, National Institute for Occupational Safety and Health, NIOSH HETA No. 2005-0135-3116.

Nolin P, Villemure R, Heroux L [2006]. Determining long-term symptoms following mild traumatic brain injury: method of interview affects self-report. Brain Inj 20(11):1147–1164.

Shoemaker RC, House DE [2005]. A time-series study of sick building syndrome: chronic, biotoxin-associated illness from exposure to water-damaged buildings. Neurotoxicol Teratol 27(1):29–46.

Shoemaker RC, House DE [2006]. Sick building syndrome and exposure to water-damaged buildings: time series study, clinical trial and mechanisms. Neurotoxicol Teratol 28(5):573–588.

Stapleton R, Mills R [2008]. Role of open-ended questionnaires in patients with balance symptoms. J Laryngol Otol 122(2):139–144.

Tranter DC, Wobbema AT, Norlien K, Dorschner DF [2009]. Indoor allergens in Minnesota schools and child care centers. J Occup Environ Hyg 6(9):582–591.

U.S. EPA [2010]. Ozone generators that are sold as air cleaners. United States Environmental Protection Agency. [http://www.epa.gov/iaq/pubs/ozonegen.html]. Date accessed: March 2011.

REFERENCES (CONTINUED)

Vesper SJ, McKinstry C, Yang C, Haugland RA, Kercsmar CM, Yike I, Schluchter MD, Kirchner HL, Sobolewski J, Allan TM, Dearborn DG [2006]. Specific molds associated with asthma. J Occup Environ Med 48(8):852–858.

Vesper S, McKinstry C, Haugland R, Wymer L, Bradham K, Ashley P, Cox D, Dewalt G, Friedman W [2007]. Development of an environmental relative moldiness index for US homes. J Occup Environ Med 49(8):829–833.

Watson D, Pennebaker JW [1989]. Health complaints, stress, and distress: Exploring the central role of negative affectivity. Psychol Rev 96(2):234–254.

Williams CW, Lees-Haley PR [1993]. Perceived toxic exposure: A review of four cognitive influences on perception of illness. J Soc Behav Pers 8(3):489–506.

Table A1. Allergens from dust samples collected on couch and office chairs

Location	Cat (Fel d1) ± CV* µg/g†	Dog (Can f1) ± CV µg/g	Dust Mite (Der f1) ± CV µg/g	Dust Mite (Der p1) ± CV µg/g
Teachers' Lounge, near Room 16— Couch	2.01 ± 0.21	2.6 ± 0.55	ND‡	ND
Room 116	4.07 ± 0.42	1.84 ± 0.39	ND	ND
Room 115	1.45 ± 0.15	0.49 ± 0.01	ND	ND
Room 129	0.61 ± 0.063	1.4 ± 0.3	ND	0.51 ± 0.13
Room 122	3.59 ± 0.37	1.27 ± 0.27	ND	ND
Room Black Box	1.37 ± 0.14	2.33 ± 0.49	ND	ND
Room 103	0.87 ± 0.09	2.1 ± 0.45	ND	ND
Room 102	0.81 ± 0.084	1.24 ± 0.26	0.49 ± 0.14	ND
Room 202	0.96 ± 0.099	1.6 ± 0.34	ND	ND
VP Front Office	1.3 ± 0.13	2.1 ± 0.45	ND	ND

No cockroach allergen was detected in any of the samples at a limit of detection of 1.6 units of allergen per gram.
*CV – Coefficient of variation
†µg/g – microgram of allergen per gram of dust
‡ND – not detected

Table A2. Fungal spore equivalents in dust, per MSQPCR and ERMI analysis

Fungal species Group 1	Room 002B*	Room 100A	Room 101*	Room 102*	Room 105*
Aspergillus flavus/oryzae	ND†	ND	ND	ND	ND
Aspergillus fumigatus	ND	1	ND	ND	ND
Aspergillus niger	1	2	ND	ND	ND
Aspergillus ochraceus	ND	ND	ND	ND	ND
Aspergillus penicillioides	4	590	ND	ND	9
Aspergillus restrictus	ND	15	ND	ND	ND
Aspergillus sclerotiorum	ND	ND	ND	ND	ND
Aspergillus sydowii	ND	ND	ND	ND	ND
Aspergillus unguis	ND	<1	ND	ND	ND
Aspergillus versicolor	ND	ND	ND	ND	ND
Aureobasidium pullulans	86	1800	ND	2200	ND
Chaetomium globosum	ND	2	ND	ND	ND
Cladosporium sphaerospermum	64	66	ND	49	ND
Eurotium (Asp.) amstelodami	1	69	ND	ND	ND
Paecilomyces variotii	ND	ND	ND	ND	ND
Penicillium brevicompactum	ND	3	ND	ND	ND
Penicillium corylophilum	ND	1	ND	ND	ND
Penicillium crustosum	ND	30	ND	ND	ND
Penicillium purpurogenum	ND	ND	ND	ND	ND
Penicillium spinulosum	ND	<1	ND	ND	6
Penicillium variabile	ND	21	ND	ND	ND
Scopulariopsis brevicaulis	ND	<1	ND	ND	ND
Scopulariopsis chartarum	1	1	ND	ND	ND
Stachybotrys chartarum	ND	ND	ND	ND	ND
Trichoderma viride	ND	ND	ND	ND	ND
Wallemia sebi	6	95	ND	ND	300
Sum of the logs, group 1	**6.02**	**16.73**	**0.00**	**5.03**	**4.21**
Group 2					
Acremonium strictum	ND	1	ND	ND	ND
Alternaria alternate	11	34	ND	ND	22
Aspergillus ustus	ND†	ND	ND	ND	ND
Cladosporium cladosporioides-1	190	970	240	300	310
Cladosporium cladosporioides-2	<1	6	ND	ND	2
Cladosporium herbarum	4	37	ND	96	ND
Epicoccum nigrum	360	340	ND	350	64
Mucor amphibiorum	1	21	ND	ND	ND
Penicillium chrysogenum	2	24	ND	ND	ND
Rhizopus stolonifer	ND	27	ND	ND	ND
Sum of the logs, group 2	**6.78**	**13.53**	**2.38**	**7.00**	**5.94**
ERMI values	**-0.76**	**3.2**	**-2.38**	**-1.97**	**-1.73**

Table A2 (continued). Fungal spore equivalents in dust, per MSQPCR and ERMI analysis

Fungal species Group 1	Room 106*	Room 107	Room 116 NS	Room 120	Room 122*
Aspergillus flavus/oryzae	ND†	ND	1	ND	ND
Aspergillus fumigatus	ND	ND	5	3	ND
Aspergillus niger	ND	ND	15	3	ND
Aspergillus ochraceus	ND	ND	4	ND	ND
Aspergillus penicillioides	ND	1	100	13	ND
Aspergillus restrictus	ND	ND	ND	ND	ND
Aspergillus sclerotiorum	ND	ND	2	ND	ND
Aspergillus sydowii	ND	ND	1	1	ND
Aspergillus unguis	ND	ND	1	ND	ND
Aspergillus versicolor	ND	ND	4	ND	ND
Aureobasidium pullulans	2100	180	5500	630	1300
Chaetomium globosum	ND	ND	5	ND	ND
Cladosporium sphaerospermum	ND	11	150	14	ND
Eurotium (Asp.) amstelodami	6	<1	43	6	ND
Paecilomyces variotii	4	1	9	ND	ND
Penicillium brevicompactum	ND	ND	29	ND	ND
Penicillium corylophilum	ND	ND	17	1	ND
Penicillium crustosum	ND	ND	17	24	ND
Penicillium purpurogenum	ND	ND	ND	ND	ND
Penicillium spinulosum	ND	ND	1	<1	ND
Penicillium variabile	ND	24	190	ND	ND
Scopulariopsis brevicaulis	ND	ND	<1	ND	ND
Scopulariopsis chartarum	ND	ND	ND	ND	ND
Stachybotrys chartarum	ND	ND	7	1	ND
Trichoderma viride	ND	ND	11	ND	ND
Wallemia sebi	30	22	330	73	ND
Sum of the logs, group 1	**6.18**	**6.02**	**25.19**	**10.04**	**4.11**
Group 2					
Acremonium strictum	ND	ND	1	ND	ND
Alternaria alternate	ND	11	110	8	ND
Aspergillus ustus	ND	ND	1	ND	ND
Cladosporium cladosporioides-1	82	190	3100	310	35
Cladosporium cladosporioides-2	<1	<1	15	2	ND
Cladosporium herbarum	ND	4	310	17	ND
Epicoccum nigrum	26	360	1000	60	ND
Mucor amphibiorum	1	1	39	3	ND
Penicillium chrysogenum	ND	2	7	11	ND
Rhizopus stolonifer	ND	ND	8	ND	ND
Sum of the logs, group 2	**3.32**	**6.78**	**15.54**	**8.22**	**1.54**
ERMI values	**2.86**	**-0.76**	**9.65**	**1.82**	**2.57**

Table A2 (continued). Fungal spore equivalents in dust, per MSQPCR and ERMI analysis

Fungal species Group 1	Room 122 NS	Room 127 NS	Room 130 NS	Boiler Room	Boiler Room
Aspergillus flavus/oryzae	ND†	ND	3	ND	ND
Aspergillus fumigatus	7	5	3	7	ND
Aspergillus niger	11	5	130	2	ND
Aspergillus ochraceus	5	ND	ND	ND	ND
Aspergillus penicillioides	21	130	6	30	44
Aspergillus restrictus	ND	ND	21	ND	ND
Aspergillus sclerotiorum	ND	23	ND	ND	ND
Aspergillus sydowii	ND	29	10	11	14
Aspergillus unguis	3	<1	<1	<1	ND
Aspergillus versicolor	2	2	2	13	5
Aureobasidium pullulans	13000	830	1600	2300	1000
Chaetomium globosum	7	ND	1	1	5
Cladosporium sphaerospermum	130	72	33	310	270
Eurotium (Asp.) amstelodami	19	1	22	8	4
Paecilomyces variotii	7	ND	ND	5	1
Penicillium brevicompactum	24	ND	9	ND	ND
Penicillium corylophilum	16	4	ND	ND	2
Penicillium crustosum	15	ND	9	ND	ND
Penicillium purpurogenum	5	ND	ND	1	ND
Penicillium spinulosum	1	ND	<1	ND	ND
Penicillium variabile	79	12	44	220	90
Scopulariopsis brevicaulis	3	ND	ND	ND	ND
Scopulariopsis chartarum	ND	ND	ND	ND	4
Stachybotrys chartarum	ND	ND	ND	150	42
Trichoderma viride	5	ND	4	ND	ND
Wallemia sebi	420	15	190	25	140
Sum of the logs, group 1	**24.05**	**14.27**	**18.95**	**18.15**	**16.84**
Group 2					
Acremonium strictum	3	ND	ND	ND	ND
Alternaria alternate	290	21	29	58	19
Aspergillus ustus	3	ND	ND	16	15
Cladosporium cladosporioides-1	6000	360	500	440	270
Cladosporium cladosporioides-2	36	3	6	2	2
Cladosporium herbarum	360	9	38	150	34
Epicoccum nigrum	3400	110	360	540	330
Mucor amphibiorum	52	1	2	4	2+
Penicillium chrysogenum	5	8	2	ND	2
Rhizopus stolonifer	5	ND	1	ND	ND
Sum of the logs, group 2	**17.97**	**8.25**	**9.68**	**11.41**	**10.74**
ERMI values	**6.08**	**6.02**	**9.27**	**6.74**	**6.10**

Table A2 (continued). Fungal spore equivalents in dust, per MSQPCR and ERMI analysis

Fungal species Group 1	Room 131 NS	Room 136	Room 142	Room 143	Room 143 NS
Aspergillus flavus/oryzae	2	ND†	ND	ND	29
Aspergillus fumigatus	4	ND	ND	3	38
Aspergillus niger	13	15	ND	ND	39
Aspergillus ochraceus	7	ND	ND	4	20
Aspergillus penicillioides	63	25	5	14	340
Aspergillus restrictus	ND	ND	ND	ND	52
Aspergillus sclerotiorum	1	ND	ND	ND	51
Aspergillus sydowii	5	ND	ND	ND	2
Aspergillus unguis	<1	ND	ND	ND	<1
Aspergillus versicolor	4	ND	ND	ND	16
Aureobasidium pullulans	5000	1300	61	1100	8400
Chaetomium globosum	3	ND	ND	ND	3
Cladosporium sphaerospermum	130	76	15	10	620
Eurotium (Asp.) amstelodami	44	ND	ND	3	360
Paecilomyces variotii	6	ND	ND	ND	10
Penicillium brevicompactum	9	59	3	ND	94
Penicillium corylophilum	4	ND	1	ND	24
Penicillium crustosum	12	ND	ND	ND	16
Penicillium purpurogenum	ND	ND	ND	ND	2
Penicillium spinulosum	<1	ND	ND	ND	1
Penicillium variabile	69	ND	ND	ND	66
Scopulariopsis brevicaulis	1	ND	<1	ND	4
Scopulariopsis chartarum	5	ND	ND	ND	9
Stachybotrys chartarum	8	ND	ND	ND	2
Trichoderma viride	3	ND	ND	ND	7
Wallemia sebi	490	ND	27	19	720
Sum of the logs, group 1	**23.91**	**9.34**	**5.58**	**8.03**	**36.37**
Group 2					
Acremonium strictum	2	ND	ND	<1	10
Alternaria alternate	120	73	11	ND	260
Aspergillus ustus	1	ND	ND	ND	ND
Cladosporium cladosporioides-1	2300	1600	180	85	12000
Cladosporium cladosporioides-2	10	6	1	<1	9
Cladosporium herbarum	180	ND	7	ND	2000
Epicoccum nigrum	1200	530	150	1	4600
Mucor amphibiorum	19	ND	2	ND	48
Penicillium chrysogenum	6	ND	1	ND	4
Rhizopus stolonifer	5	ND	2	ND	3
Sum of the logs, group 2	**14.84**	**8.56**	**6.93**	**1.93**	**17.74**
ERMI values	**9.07**	**0.78**	**-1.35**	**6.10**	**18.63**

Table A2 (continued). Fungal spore equivalents in dust, per MSQPCR and ERMI analysis

Fungal species Group 1	Room 210 NS	Room 211 NS	Room 213 NS	Room 217 NS
Aspergillus flavus/oryzae	3	<1	4	2
Aspergillus fumigates	2	4	3	4
Aspergillus niger	18	44	18	140
Aspergillus ochraceus	ND†	5	4	ND
Aspergillus penicillioides	15	23	17	15
Aspergillus restrictus	22	31	ND	ND
Aspergillus sclerotiorum	2	1	2	ND
Aspergillus sydowii	2	25	3	2
Aspergillus unguis	ND	1	<1	1
Aspergillus versicolor	ND	2	2	2
Aureobasidium pullulans	5300	7000	2600	6800
Chaetomium globosum	6	33	3	2
Cladosporium sphaerospermum	81	58	51	64
Eurotium (Asp.) amstelodami	23	19	11	7
Paecilomyces variotii	13	11	3	3
Penicillium brevicompactum	6	10	7	23
Penicillium corylophilum	4	4	2	4
Penicillium crustosum	6	14	7	15
Penicillium purpurogenum	ND	ND	1	1
Penicillium spinulosum	<1	1	<1	1
Penicillium variabile	16	10	13	27
Scopulariopsis brevicaulis	<1	1	<1	<1
Scopulariopsis chartarum	ND	1	ND	1
Stachybotrys chartarum	22	2	1	ND
Trichoderma viride	4	1	1	ND
Wallemia sebi	390	170	100	88
Sum of the logs, group 1	**21.93**	**23.22**	**17.48**	**18.61**
Group 2				
Acremonium strictum	<1	1	<1	2
Alternaria alternate	140	160	70	140
Aspergillus ustus	2	34	ND	7
Cladosporium cladosporioides-1	1100	1500	1200	1700
Cladosporium cladosporioides-2	13	62	25	14
Cladosporium herbarum	390	290	220	240
Epicoccum nigrum	100	1300	610	1700
Mucor amphibiorum	18	23	18	10
Penicillium chrysogenum	14	14	7	4
Rhizopus stolonifer	47	<1	4	<1
Sum of the logs, group 2	**16.27**	**16.78**	**14.17**	**14.89**
ERMI values	**5.66**	**6.44**	**3.31**	**3.72**

*low sample weight
†ND = not detected

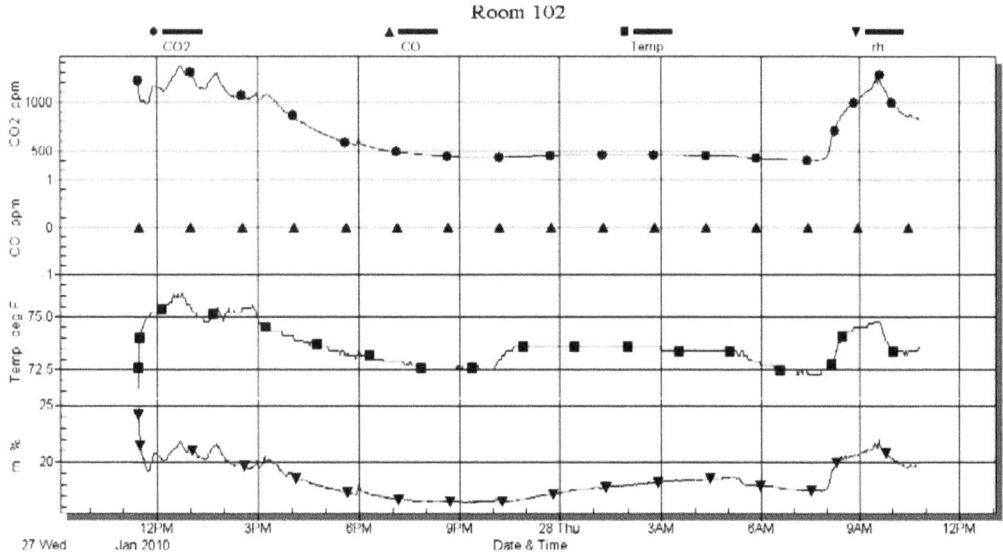

Figure A1. Graph of CO_2, CO, Temperature, and RH for Room 102.

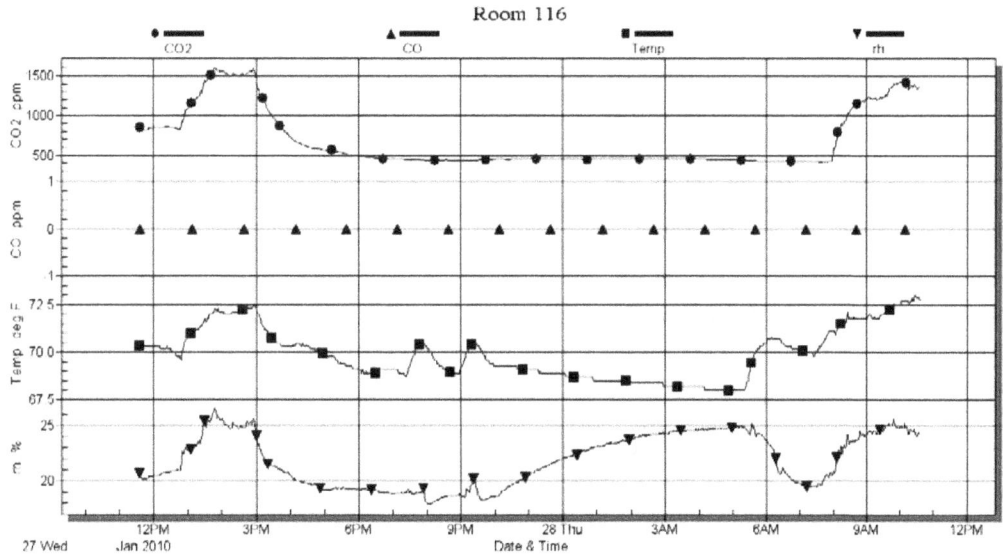

Figure A2. Graph of CO_2, CO, Temperature, and RH for Room 116.

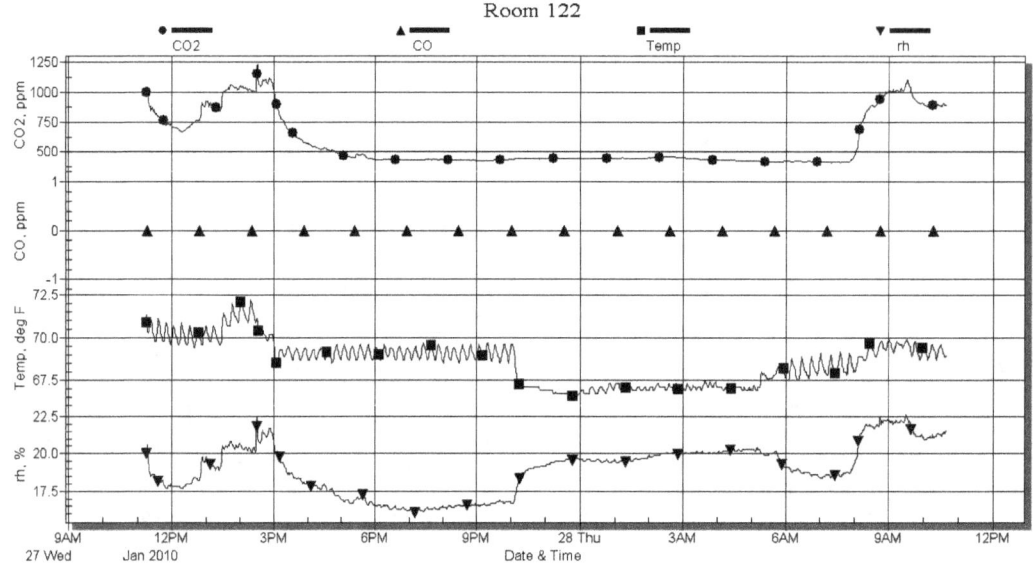

Figure A3. Graph of CO_2, CO, Temperature, and RH for Room 122.

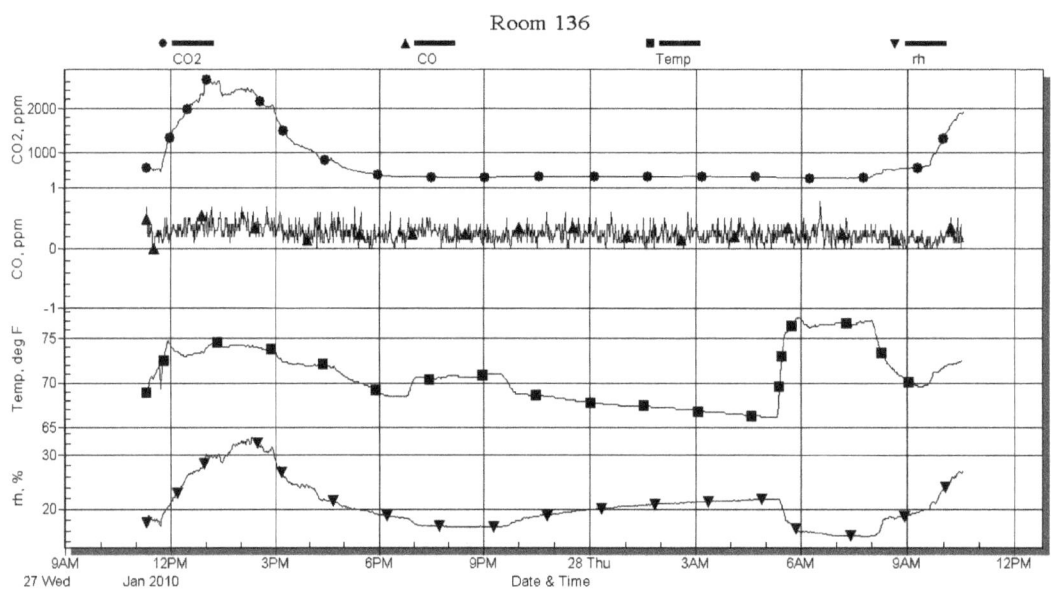

Figure A4. Graph of CO_2, CO, Temperature, and RH for Room 136.

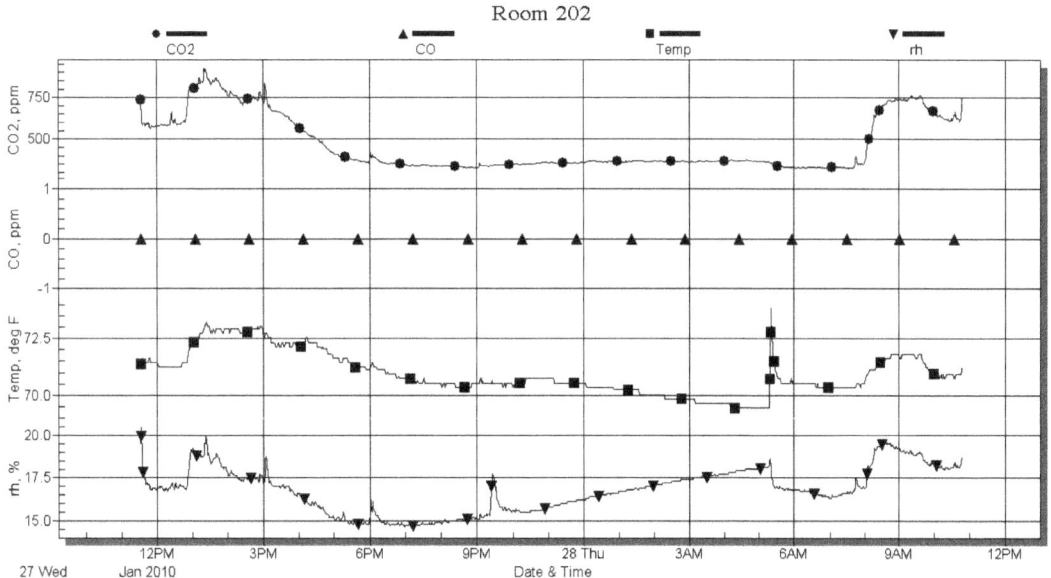

Figure A5. Graph of CO_2, CO, Temperature, and RH for Room 202.

Microbial Contamination

Exposure to microbes is not unique to the indoor environment. No environment, indoors or out, is completely free from microbes, not even a surgical operating room. Remediation of microbial contamination may improve IEQ conditions even though a specific cause-effect relationship is not determined. NIOSH investigators routinely recommend the remediation of observed microbial contamination and the correction of situations that are favorable for microbial growth and bioaerosol dissemination.

Mold

The types and severity of symptoms related to exposure to mold in the indoor environment depend in part on the extent of the mold present, the extent of the individual's exposure, and the susceptibility of the individual (for example, whether they have preexisting allergies or asthma). In general, excessive exposure to fungi may produce health problems by several primary mechanisms, including allergy or hypersensitivity, infection, and toxic effects. Additionally, molds produce a variety of VOCs, the most common of which is ethanol, that have been postulated to cause upper-airway irritation. However, as discussed above, potential irritant effects of VOCs from exposure to mold in the indoor environment are not well understood. Evidence also shows that exposure to fungal fragments that can contain allergens, toxins, and $(1\rightarrow3)$-β-D-glucan may occur [Górney et al. 2002; Brasel et al. 2005; Reponen et al. 2006].

Allergic responses are the most common type of health problem associated with exposure to molds. These health problems may include sneezing; itching of the nose, eyes, mouth, or throat; nasal stuffiness and runny nose; and red, itchy eyes. Repeated or single exposure to mold or mold spores may cause previously nonsensitized individuals to become sensitized. Molds can trigger asthma symptoms (shortness of breath, wheezing, cough) in persons who are allergic to mold. In the 2004 report, "Damp Indoor Spaces and Health," the IOM found sufficient evidence of an association between mold or dampness indoors and nasal and throat symptoms, asthma symptoms in sensitized asthmatics, wheeze, cough, and hypersensitivity pneumonitis in susceptible persons [IOM 2004]. The IOM found limited or suggestive evidence of an association between lower respiratory illness in healthy children and damp indoor spaces. There was inadequate or insufficient evidence to determine whether an association exists between damp indoor spaces and dyspnea, airflow obstruction in healthy persons, mucous membrane irritation, skin symptoms, chronic obstructive pulmonary disease, asthma development, inhalation fevers in nonoccupational settings, fatigue, cancer, reproductive effects, neuropsychiatric effects, lower respiratory illness in healthy adults, gastrointestinal problems, rheumatologic or immune problems, or acute idiopathic pulmonary hemorrhage in infants. No health conditions met the level of evidence for causation. In 2009, WHO published guidelines for protection of public health from mold and other exposures in damp buildings [WHO 2009]. Based on its review of the scientific literature for this report, the WHO concluded that there was sufficient epidemiological evidence that occupants of damp buildings are at risk of developing upper and lower respiratory tract symptoms (including cough, wheeze, and dyspnea), respiratory infections, asthma, and exacerbation of asthma. The WHO also concluded that limited evidence suggests associations between bronchitis and allergic rhinitis and damp buildings. They noted clinical evidence that exposure to mold and other microbial agents in damp buildings is associated with hypersensitivity pneumonitis.

People with weakened immune systems (immune-compromised or immune-suppressed individuals) may be more vulnerable to infections by molds. For example, Aspergillus fumigatus is a fungal species that has been found almost everywhere on every conceivable type of substrate. It has been known to infect the lungs of immune-compromised individuals after inhalation of the airborne spores [Wald and Stave 1994; Brandt et al. 2006]. Healthy individuals are usually not vulnerable to infections from airborne mold exposure.

No exposure guidelines for mold in air exist, so it is not possible to distinguish between "safe" and "unsafe" levels of exposure. Nevertheless, the potential for health problems is an important reason to prevent indoor mold growth and to remediate any indoor mold contamination. Moisture intrusion, along with nutrient sources such as building materials or furnishings, allows mold to grow indoors, so it is important to keep the building interior and furnishings dry. NIOSH concurs with the U.S. EPA's recommendations to remedy mold contamination in indoor environments ([http://www.epa.gov/iaq/molds/mold_remediation.html) [Redd SC 2002; US EPA 2001]. Additional information on health effects and mold remediation can be found in the Centers for Disease Control and Prevention document *Mold Prevention Strategies and Possible Health Effects in the Aftermath of Hurricanes and Major Floods* (http://www.cdc.gov/mmwr/preview/ mmwrhtml/ rr5508a1.htm).

Standards specific to the nonindustrial indoor environment do not exist. Measurement of indoor environmental contaminants has seldom proved helpful in determining the cause of symptoms, except where there are unusual sources or a proven relationship between specific exposures and disease. With few exceptions, concentrations of frequently measured chemical substances in the indoor work environment fall well below the recommended OELs published by NIOSH [NIOSH 2005], ACGIH [ACGIH 2010], and AIHA [AIHA 2010], as well as the mandatory PELs set by OSHA [29 CFR 1910 (general industry)]. ANSI/ASHRAE has published recommended building ventilation and thermal comfort guidelines [ANSI/ASHRAE 2010a; ANSI/ASHRAE 2010b]. The ACGIH and AIHA have also developed a manual of guidelines for approaching investigations of building-related symptoms that might be caused by airborne living organisms or their effluents [ACGIH 1999; AIHA 2008]. Other resources that provide guidance for establishing acceptable IEQ are available through U.S. EPA at http://www.epa.gov/iaq, especially the U.S. EPA *Indoor Air Quality Tools for Schools* (http://www.epa.gov/iaq/schools/) and the joint U.S. EPA/NIOSH document *Building Air Quality, A Guide for Building Owners and Facility Managers* (http://www.epa. gov/iaq/largebldgs/baqtoc.html).

Heating, Ventilating, and Air-Conditioning

One of the most common deficiencies in the indoor environment is the improper operation and maintenance of ventilation systems and other building components [Rosenstock 1996]. NIOSH investigators have found that correcting HVAC problems often reduces reported symptoms. The majority of studies of ventilation rates and building occupant symptoms have shown that rates below 10 Ls^{-1}/person (which equates to 20 CFM per person) are associated with one or more health symptoms [Seppanen et al. 1999]. Moreover, higher ventilation rates, from 10 Ls^{-1}/person up to 20 Ls^{-1}/person, have been associated with further significant decreases in the prevalence of symptoms [Seppanen et al. 1999]. Thus, improved HVAC operation and maintenance, higher ventilation rates, and comfortable temperature and RH can all potentially serve to improve symptoms without ever identifying any specific cause-effect relationships. When conducting an IEQ evaluation, NIOSH investigators often measure ventilation and comfort indicators, such as CO_2, temperature, and RH, to provide information relative to the functioning and control of HVAC systems.

Carbon Dioxide

CO_2 is a normal constituent of exhaled breath and is not considered a building air pollutant. It can be used as an indicator of whether sufficient quantities of outdoor air are being introduced into an occupied space for acceptable odor control. However, CO_2 is not an effective indicator of ventilation adequacy if the ventilated area is not occupied at its usual occupant density at the time the CO_2 is measured. ASHRAE notes in an informative appendix to standard 62.1 that indoor CO_2 concentrations no greater than 700 ppm above outdoor CO_2 concentrations will satisfy a substantial majority (about 80%) of visitors with regard to odor from sedentary building occupants (body odor) [ANSI/ASHRAE 2010b]. Elevated CO_2 concentrations suggest that other indoor contaminants may also be increased. If CO_2 concentrations are elevated, the amount of outdoor air introduced into the ventilated space may need to be increased. When CO_2 concentrations are used as an indicator to determine outdoor air requirements, ventilation system designs that rely on duct-mounted CO_2 sensors should have some form of ventilation efficiency documentation that relates concentration values observed at the duct location with those observed within the breathing zone of the occupied space.

Temperature and Relative Humidity

Temperature and RH measurements are often collected as part of an IEQ evaluation because these parameters affect the perception of comfort in an indoor environment. The perception of thermal comfort is related to one's metabolic heat production, the transfer of heat to the environment, physiological adjustments, and body temperature [NIOSH 1986]. Heat transfer from the body to the environment is influenced by factors such as temperature, humidity, air movement, personal activities, and clothing. The ANSI/ASHRAE Standard 55-2010, Thermal Environmental Conditions for Human Occupancy, specifies conditions in which 80% or more of the occupants would be expected to find the environment thermally acceptable [ANSI/ASHRAE 2010a]. Assuming slow air movement and 50% RH, the operative temperatures recommended by

ANSI/ASHRAE range from 68.5°F to 76°F in the winter, and from 75°F to 80.5°F in the summer. The difference between the two is largely due to seasonal clothing selection. ANSI/ASHRAE also recommends that RH be maintained at or below 65% [ANSI/ASHRAE 2010a]. Excessive humidity can promote the excessive growth of microorganisms and dust mites.

References

ACGIH [1999]. Bioaerosols: assessment and control. Cincinnati, OH: American Conference of Governmental Industrial Hygienists.

ACGIH [2010]. 2010 TLVs® and BEIs®: threshold limit values for chemical substances and physical agents and biological exposure indices. Cincinnati, OH: American Conference of Governmental Industrial Hygienists.

AIHA [2008]. Recognition, evaluation, and control of indoor mold. Prezant B, Weekes DM, Miller JD eds. Fairfax, VA: American Industrial Hygiene Association.

AIHA [2010]. 2010 Emergency response planning guidelines (ERPG) & workplace environmental exposure levels (WEEL) handbook. Fairfax, VA: American Industrial Hygiene Association.

ANSI/ASHRAE [2010a]. Thermal environmental conditions for human occupancy. American National Standards Institute/ASHRAE standard 55-2010. Atlanta, GA: American Society for Heating, Refrigerating, and Air-Conditioning Engineers, Inc.

ANSI/ASHRAE [2010b]. Ventilation for acceptable indoor air quality. American National Standards Institute/ASHRAE standard 62.1-2010. Atlanta, GA: American Society of Heating, Refrigerating, and Air-Conditioning Engineers, Inc.

Brandt M, Brown C, Burkhart J, Burton N, Cox-Ganser J, Damon S, Falk H, Fridkin S, Garbe P, McGeehin M, Morgan J, Page E, Rao C, Redd S, Sinks T, Trout D, Wallingford K, Warnock D, Weissman D [2006]. Mold prevention strategies and possible health effects in the aftermath of hurricanes and major floods. MMWR 55(RR-8):1–27.

Brasel TL, Martin JM, Carriker CG, Wilson SC, Straus DC [2005]. Detection of airborne Stachybotrys chartarum macrocyclic trichothecene mycotoxins in the indoor environment. Appl Environ Microbiol 71(11):7376–7388.

CFR. Code of Federal Regulations. Washington, DC: U.S. Government Printing Office, Office of the Federal Register.

Górny RL, Reponen T, Willeke K, Schmechel D, Robine E, Boissier M, Grinshpun SA [2002]. Fungal fragments as indoor air biocontaminants. Appl Environ Microbiol 68(7):3522–3531.

IOM [2004]. Human health effects associated with damp indoor environments. In: Damp indoor spaces and health. Institute of Medicine, National Academy Press, Washington, DC. pp. 183–269.

NIOSH [1986]. Criteria for a recommended standard: occupational exposure to hot environments, revised criteria. Cincinnati, OH: U.S. Department of Health and Human Services, Centers for Disease Control, National Institute for Occupational Safety and Health, DHHS (NIOSH) Publication No. 86-13.

NIOSH [2005]. NIOSH pocket guide to chemical hazards. Cincinnati, OH: U.S. Department of Health and Human Services, Centers for Disease Control and Prevention, National Institute for Occupational Safety and Health, DHHS (NIOSH) Publication No. 2005-149. [http://www.cdc.gov/niosh/npg/]. Date accessed: March 2011.

Redd SC [2002]. State of the science on molds and human health. Statement for the Record Before the Subcommittee on Oversight and Investigations and Housing and Community Opportunity, Committee on Financial Services, United States House of Representatives. Atlanta, GA: U.S. Department of Health and Human Services, Centers for Disease Control and Prevention.

Reponen T, Seo S-C, Iossifova Y, Adhikari A, Grinshpun SA [2006]. New field-compatible method for collection and analysis of β-glucan in fungal fragments. Abstracts of the International Aerosol Conference, St. Paul, Minnesota, p. 955.

Rosenstock L [1996]. NIOSH Testimony to the U.S. Department of Labor on indoor air quality. Applied Occupational and Environmental Hygiene 11(12):1365-1370.

Seppanen OA, Fisk WJ, Mendell MJ [1999]. Association of ventilation rates and CO2 concentrations with health and other responses in commercial and institutional buildings. Indoor Air 9(4):226-252.

U.S. EPA [2001]. Mold remediation in schools and commercial buildings. Washington, DC: United States Environmental Protection Agency, Office of Air and Radiation, Indoor Environments Division. EPA Publication No. 402-K-01-001.

Wald P, Stave G [1994]. Fungi. In: Physical and biological hazards of the workplace. New York: Van Nostrand Reinhold, p. 394.

WHO [2009]. WHO guidelines for indoor air quality: dampness and mould. Geneva, Switzerland: World Health Organization. [http://www.euro.who.int/document/e92645.pdf]. Date accessed: March 2011.

This page left intentionally blank

The Hazard Evaluations and Technical Assistance Branch (HETAB) of the National Institute for Occupational Safety and Health (NIOSH) conducts field investigations of possible health hazards in the workplace. These investigations are conducted under the authority of Section 20(a)(6) of the Occupational Safety and Health Act of 1970, 29 U.S.C. 669(a)(6), which authorizes the Secretary of Health and Human Services, following a written request from any employer or authorized representative of employees, to determine whether any substance normally found in the place of employment has potentially toxic effects in such concentrations as used or found. HETAB also provides, upon request, technical and consultative assistance to federal, state, and local agencies; labor; industry; and other groups or individuals to control occupational health hazards and to prevent related trauma and disease.

The findings and conclusions in this report are those of the authors and do not necessarily represent the views of NIOSH. Mention of any company or product does not constitute endorsement by NIOSH. In addition, citations to websites external to NIOSH do not constitute NIOSH endorsement of the sponsoring organizations or their programs or products. Furthermore, NIOSH is not responsible for the content of these websites. All Web addresses referenced in this document were accessible as of the publication date.

This report was prepared by Elena Page, Nancy Burton, Melody Kawamoto, and R. Todd Niemeier of HETAB, Division of Surveillance, Hazard Evaluations and Field Studies. Analytical support was provided by Steven Vesper, United States Environmental Protection Agency, National Exposure Research Laboratory, Cincinnati, Ohio, and EmLabs P&K, Cherry Hill, New Jersey. Health communication assistance was provided by Stefanie Evans. Editorial assistance was provided by Seleen Collins. Desktop publishing was performed by Greg Hartle.

Copies of this report have been sent to employee and management representatives at the middle school, the state health department, and the Occupational Safety and Health Administration Regional Office. This report is not copyrighted and may be freely reproduced. The report may be viewed and printed at http://www.cdc.gov/niosh/hhe/. Copies may be purchased from the National Technical Information Service at 5825 Port Royal Road, Springfield, Virginia 22161.

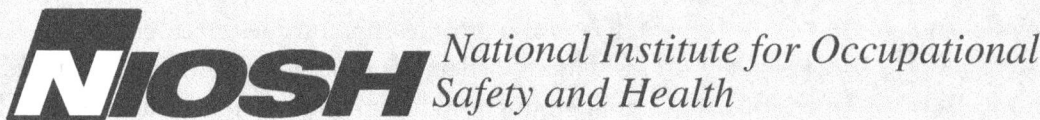
National Institute for Occupational Safety and Health

Delivering on the Nation's promise: Safety and health at work for all people through research and prevention.

To receive NIOSH documents or information about occupational safety and health topics, contact NIOSH at:

1-800-CDC-INFO (1-800-232-4636)

TTY: 1-888-232-6348

E-mail: cdcinfo@cdc.gov

or visit the NIOSH web site at: **www.cdc.gov/niosh.**

For a monthly update on news at NIOSH, subscribe to NIOSH eNews by visiting **www.cdc.gov/niosh/eNews.**

SAFER • HEALTHIER • PEOPLE™

www.ingramcontent.com/pod-product-compliance
Lightning Source LLC
Chambersburg PA
CBHW080911290526
45795CB00007BA/2491